Gua Sha

Practical Guide to Unlock the Secret Of Modern Beauty By Fighting The Signs Of Aging Naturally Along-with a Healthy Immune System, Natural Face-lift and Skin

Adams T. David

Table of Contents

Introduction

Are you aware of the fact that Gua-sha is supposed to handle stagnant energy, called *chi*; professionals believe that this *"chi"* is responsible for swellings in any part of the body; swelling is the reason behind several conditions associated with chronic pain. Massaging the skin's surface is considered to help split up this energy, reduce irritation, and promote recovery.

As many out there will ask, what's the true definition of Gua-sha? Gua-sha is a part of traditional Chinese medication (TCM); it can also be known as "scraping," "spooning," or "coining." It is professionally used as an instrument to scrape people's pores and skin; it is said to have a therapeutic advantage. The procedure of this particular medication has a French name called *tribo-effleurage*. Gua-sha is an all-natural option therapy that involves scraping your skin layer with a therapeutic massage tool to boost your blood circulation. This ancient Chinese curing technique provides a unique method of better health and also dealing with issues like chronic pain.

In gua-sha, a technician scrapes your skin layer with brief or long strokes to stimulate microcirculation of the smooth cells, which increases blood circulation; they make these strokes with a smooth-edged device known as a *Gua-therapeutic massage tool*, the specialist applies massage essential oil to your skin layer, and then uses the tool to scrape your skin layer in a downward movement frequently.

Where can this be performed? Always note that Gua-sha is usually performed on the back, buttocks, neck, hands, and legs; a mild version from it is even applied to the facial skin as a cosmetic technique. Your specialist may apply moderate pressure, and steadily increase strength to regulate how much pressure you are designed for.

I heartily congratulate you for getting your hands on this book which encompasses details of what you could ask for or need in this guide.

Chapter 1

What is Face Gua Sha?

Face Gua-Sha could be a well-known scraping massage technique made by Traditional Chinese Medicine; it started as a remedy done exclusively on your own body to boost blood circulation, move lymphatic stagnation, and releases muscle tension. After a while, a much gentler version was designed for the facial skin, that involves a light gliding motion tone, lift, and smoothens your skin layer. Tools of assorted shapes made of crystal (such as for example jade or Rose quartz) are found in mixture with light pressure in an upward and outward movement.

The target is to de-puff the facial skin by facilitating lymphatic drainage in to the neck and bring fresh blood & nutrients to your skin layer for the healthy glow. As you softly scrape your skin layer, micro-circulation is usually improved, which carries oxygenated bloodstream towards the dermal layers clearing congestion, stimulating cell renewal, and brightening your appearance. This hurry of blood brings nutrients that produce cell regeneration and tissues repair far more productive, which is incredibly helpful if you're coping with acne or wanting to eliminate acne scarring.

Overall, it's an amazingly easy addition to your early morning or evening epidermis routine that demands 5 minutes and will give you noticeable lift and shine every time.

Gua-Sha Tools

Long-time ago, Gua-Sha scraping tools were made of things such as for example bone and even cow horns. I used to be once told that's because cow horns are excellent conductors of vigour, as cows use their horns to communicate; whether that's true or not, I have no thought, although I'd want to trust the idea of telepathic cows. Irrespective, it's wise that crystals are used today because they're also considered to emit energy.

ADVANTAGES OF Gua-Sha

Cosmetic Gua-Sha movement is a lymphatic liquid that gets built-up in the facial skin, which bears away poisons that may contribute to acne and boring, irritated skin.

Gua-Sha benefits include:

· Shades the muscles from the facial skin that may assist with sagging skin

· Companies and hydrates your skin layer

· Relaxes muscle stress in the facial skin, increasing full-body stress alleviation (puts the body inside a parasympathetic condition, which is wonderful for those who which has trouble drifting off to sleep)

· Boosts blood flow & circulation

· Moves stagnant bloodstream that plays a component in dark circles & under-eye bags.

· Helps your skin layer overcome blemishes & acne scars

· Prevents lines and wrinkles and helps clean existing lines

· De-puffs and slims the facial skin

· Instantly lifts and plumps your skin layer

· Allows serums to penetrate deeper post-treatment

· Aids throat pain & headaches because of tight muscle or fascia.

How exactly to Perform Gua-Sha in the home

If you wish to begin in the throat/jaw first and work your path up, and that means you beginning lymphatic drainage at the least expensive stage; that way, when you get up to your forehead and vision area, the liquid and poisons have some place to drain into as being a funnel.

Additionally, you intend to use very light pressure; if your skin layer begins to get very red, it's to company rather than concentrating on the lymph. Lymph needs light-weight because your lymphatic vessels are so near the top. Your tools ought to be angled at about 15-20°, almost smooth to your skin layer in order that you're not stabbing yourself and will experience the soft pull that plays a component in the lifting impact.

Always scrape towards outer sides from the facial skin and sweep down for the guts when you're doing all of your neck, meaning your lymph drains appropriately in to the nodes above your collarbone.

How come Lymphatic Drainage is Important?

Do you realize your lymphatic system is doubly significant as your circulatory system? While your circulatory system has your center to pump and clean your bloodstream automatically, your lymph doesn't have any built-in pump whatsoever. Lymph just goes on hand through exercise, massage therapy, and diet, which is why it's straightforward to get supported by this modern lifestyle.

The lymphatic system was not fully understood under western culture until significantly less than 2 decades ago - yet ancient systems of medicine such as for example TCM or Ayurveda view is probably the first places to consider stagnation whenever your person is ill. The

AMA historically ignores lymph stagnation as grounds behind disease, whereas other countries such as for example Germany use specific Lymphatic Drainage techniques as an end to fibrocystic breast disease, allergies, persistent sinusitis, arthritis, eczema, coronary disease and more.

An indicator that your lymphatic system is usually sluggish is:

·   If your body is usually a residence, think about your blood as the tap as well as your lymph as the drains: As I said, your bloodstream is always pumping, meaning your valves are continually operating. The problem is that they run straight into the region that isn't nonetheless assured to visit. When particles from your bloodstream are too large to become removed from your liver organ, kidneys, or epidermis, it goes straight into your lymphatic vessels. So when those "drains" aren't moving correctly, stagnation and disease occur.

The most typical causes of poor lymphatic circulation are:

·   Stress - The chemistry of stress is degenerative and lymph-congesting in character. Overwork and insufficient rest periods bargain your lymph, digestion of food, and liver organ Qi.

· Digestive Imbalances - Irritation from the intestinal villi credited to inflammatory foods and poor digestion congests us because almost all your lymph surrounds the gut via "Gut Associated Lymph Tissue" (GALT). Discover my post here about 11 uncommon (yet straightforward) methods to increase your digestion. To obtain additional in-depth solutions, I've another post here that clarifies the four main causes of poor digestion and just how to address most of them.

· Deficiencies - Nutrient deficiencies, especially iodine, impact the lymph. Iodine really helps to mitigate the results of the harmful environment (hello pesticide-sprayed world!) and supports the lymph at a mobile level. See my post here on advantages of seaweed.

· Emotional/Religious - Shame, blocked circulation of pleasure in life, depression, repressed emotions.

· Insufficient Activity - Since I explained that this

lymph doesn't have any pump, this will depend upon you to accomplish it; an inactive lifestyle/working a table job seriously compromises lymphatic flow.

· Diet - Foods can either help or avoid the blast of lymph. Most unfortunate: prepared/packaged, processed sugars (corn syrup), white flour.

Face Gua-Sha is one small section of the lymphatic puzzle, nonetheless it will help to get things moving, especially if you possess chronic issues with mucus build-up within your sinuses.

Actions you may take to improve lymphatic blood flow include:

· Take strolls day-by-day, especially after foods (even for ten minutes).

· Eat the white section of the orange! (click that for my post upon this concern).

· Consume red-staining foods (pure cranberry juice, blueberries, and raspberries).

· Decrease the time frame that you sit back each day give dry-brushing a join a rebounder for just a few minutes, many times per daytime.

Chapter 2

Uses of Gua-sha

Listed here are various ways of gua-sha meditation technique:

·   Gua-sha is generally used to ease muscle and joint pain; conditions from the muscles and bone tissue are referred to as musculoskeletal disorders; several examples include backwards pain, tendon stress, and carpal tunnel symptoms.

·   Practitioners declare that gua-sha also offers the benefit of disease-fighting capability and reduced amount of irritation. Sometimes, gua-sha is useful to look after a chilly, fever, or problems with the lungs.

·   Small injuries to the body, just like the bruises due to gua-sha, are now and again referred to as micro-trauma; these produce a reply in the body that might help separate scar tissue formation. Micro-trauma also can help with fibrosis, which can be an accumulation of an excessive amount of connective tissue whenever your body heals.

· Physiotherapists might use IASTM on connective cells that aren't wanting to move bones since it will; this problem could be credited to repetitive stress damage or another condition. Gua-sha could be used alongside other treatments, such as for example extending and conditioning exercises.

Great things about Gua-Sha

Researchers have completed small studies on another sets of individuals to learn if gua-sha works:

· Women near menopause.

· People using the guitar and also helps to relieve pain from the neck of computer users.

· Male weightlifters, to aid with recovery after training.

· Old adults with back pain.

· Women found that pre-menopausal symptoms, such as for example perspiration, insomnia, and headaches, were reduced after gua-sha.

A 2014 study found that gua-sha improved the amount of motion and reduced pain in individuals who used personal computers frequently. Also, another research in 2017 demonstrates weightlifters that had gua-sha experience found it better to lift weight after treatment.

Old adults with back pain were treated with either gua-sha or a hot pack; both treatments relieved symptoms similarly well; however, the effects of gua-sha lasted a lot longer. After weekly, those that had received gua-sha treatment reported greater versatility and less back pain compared to the other group.

UNWANTED SIDE EFFECTS and Risks

Gua-sha often burst tiny arteries near to the surface of your skin layer called capillaries. It generates the distinctive red or crimson bruises, referred to as sha. The injuries usually have a few days or weeks to heal and may exist tender while healing, people might take an over-the-counter painkiller, such as for example ibuprofen, to aid with pain and reduce bloating. A person should protect the bruised region and become mindful of never bumping it (applying a snowpack might help reduce swelling and simply any pain).

Gua-sha professionals shouldn't break your skin layer through the procedure, but there are a risk it could happen; broken pores and surface escalates the possibility of illness, so a gua-sha specialist should sterilize their tools between treatments.

Gua-sha isn't perfect for everybody; people who shouldn't possess gua-sha consist of those:

·   Who own medical ailments inside your skin or veins?

·   Who bleed very easily.

·   Who take medication to thin their blood.

·   Who've deep vein thrombosis?

·   Who experience contamination, tumor, or wound

that hasn't healed fully.

· Who comes with an implant, just like a pacemaker or internal defibrillator.

Is Gua-Sha Painful?

Treatment isn't reported to be painful, but gua-sha deliberately causes bruising, which can cause discomfort for a number of people; these bruises should heal in just a few days.

Gua-Sha Tools and Technique

Gua-sha equipment

A handheld tool with curved edges is employed in gua-sha. Typically, a spoon or coin will be employed to scrape your skin layer; however, in modern practice, therapists use just a little, hand-held tool with rounded edges.

Gua-sha tools have a tendency to end up being weighted to greatly help the specialist doing the duty to usage pressure.

Professionals of traditional East Asian medication see some materials as using a power that may support recovery - these materials include bian-rock, jade, and rose quartz. Medical quality stainless is often utilized for IASTM or when gua-sha is conducted in an infirmary. Professionals will apply gas to the spot of the body that is treated, that allows the therapist to utilize the tool over the skin more efficiently. The gua-sha practitioner will press these devices in to the body with smooth, firm strokes in one path; if Gua-sha continues to be completed around the trunk or back from the legs, a person may need to lay face down on a massage therapy table.

Chapter 3

Gua-Sha Materials: Comprehensive

Check out our list below and that means you can see the very best materials to consider:

1.   Bian Stone

Bian stones are thought to be the very best tools for gua-sha because they have probably the most ultrasonic pulses and the very best collection of frequency. Using Bian stones for therapeutic is centuries-old. In the "Nei Jing," a historical Chinese Medical publication, it lists "acupuncture, moxibustion, natural medication, Qigong, and Bian rock therapy" as the five primary medical ways of the "Yellow Emperor," a deity in Chinese religious beliefs. What's impressive is that Bian rock therapy predates acupuncture.

If you want to do Gua-Sha the authentic way, use Bian rocks.

2.   Jade

Jade is our second best pick for gua-sha devices. It is known to possess qi energy that's nearly exactly like the qi vigour of your body. Therefore, it really is ideal for healing treatments. In the olden times, barefoot doctors in China cannot afford traditional gua-sha tools, so they got scraps from jade carvers and used them as gua-sha tools. Today, jade is still widely used as a result of this healing technique.

3.   Buffalo Horn

Genuine Bian rocks derive from the city of Sibin in China. If you are desperate for Bian rocks to use, Buffalo horn is another excellent option.

In Chinese medicine, a buffalo horn includes a chilly property and an acrid/salty flavor. The acridity enhances qi and blood circulation, nourishes, and moistens. The saltiness, alternatively, relaxes tightness and softens hardness. Finally, the coldness dispels warmth and eliminates poisons in the body.

While American buffalo are from your endangered list;

in the event that you worry about where buffalo horns are derived from, obtain jade, natural stone, or steel instead.

4.   Stainless Steel

Medical-grade stainless tools certainly are a favorite choice for DASCM (Device Assisted Soft Cells Mobilization) and so are only a modern development of Gua-Sha. If you want newer materials, you are able to consider Stainless and even Titanium implements.

5.   Rose Quartz

Rose quartz is considered to open up the guts chakra and reduce pressure in the guts. It is a pleasant stone that may be found in a delicate red colorization.

Just like a Gua-Sha tool, it really is smooth and an excellent weight; others though believe that it is hard to carry and pick the buffalo horn or bian rock. Any object - as being a coin, a spoon, or a cover - can be employed for Gua-Sha. Acquiring the best apply, though, makes the entire experience convenient and, with techniques, even more memorable as you utilize tools that become special for you personally.

Like this of a historical type of recovery, you'll exist managing your stress and diseases in more natural ways instead of relying on pharmaceuticals or higher vices that only bring short-term alleviation.

Gua Sha Jade Stone

Gua-Sha for the facial skin and neck is known as the Eastern Botox or Eastern Facelift for grounds; this Traditional Chinese medication treatment, when placed on the facial skin, gets the next results:

-        Companies up your sagging face muscles

-        Smoothens your skin layer and reduces the looks of lines and wrinkles on your face

-        Improves dark circles and eyebags beneath the eye (the sort you get from advancing generation)

-        Lightens   age   places   and   other   epidermis discolorations

-        Your tone gets rosier and more radiant

\- Helps remove acne, rosacea, and additional epidermis diseases on your face.

How to use:

Our Rose Quartz Gua-Sha tools include a printed beginner's guide to obtain the most from it in the home.

Konjac Face Sponge - Pure

Perfect for everyone, a 100% Pure Konjac Sponge deeply cleanses, eliminates blackheads and gently exfoliates your skin layer. The initial online like framework from the veggie fibers really helps to stimulate blood flow and promote epidermis cell renewal.

How to use:

Before use, constantly wash the sponge thoroughly. We recommend plunging it in normal water and squeezing it often. If the sponge offers dry, ever allow it fully absorb water before putting it against your skin layer.

Softly massage the facial skin and body inside a circular motion around to exfoliate dead skin cells and deep cleanse. The massaging will stimulate exhausted epidermis & encourage epidermis renewal. Soap or cleansing solution could be placed into the sponge if desired but isn't essential.

Your sponge should last almost a year, but once it begins to look tired, or begins to breakdown. Please replace it. The better treatment you consider of the sponge, the lot longer it'll last.

Konjac Face Sponge - Bamboo Charcoal

Filled with nutrient-rich triggered carbon, the Konjac Sponge with Bamboo Charcoal deep cleans pores to eliminate blackheads and dirt and grime while absorbing extra oils and toxins. An all-natural antioxidant, it kills persistent acne-causing bacteria, which is an efficient natural treatment for acne victims.

How to use:

Before use, perpetually wash the sponge thoroughly. We recommend plunging it in normal water and squeezing it often. If the sponge offers dry out, allow it to fully absorb water before putting it against your skin layer.

Lightly massage the facial skin and body within a circular motion around, to exfoliate dead skin cells, and deeply cleanse; the massaging will stimulate exhausted epidermis & encourage epidermis renewals Soap or cleansing solution could be placed into the sponge if desired but isn't essential.

Your sponge should last almost a year, but once it begins to look tired, or begins to breakdown. Please replace it. The better treatment you consider of the sponge, the lot longer it'll last.

Konjac Face Sponge - GREEN TEA HERB

GREEN TEA EXTRACT herb is naturally filled up with antioxidants which have a cell-protecting function; they own a considerable antioxidant impact that protects your skin layer through the damaging effect of free radicals. This natural component includes a softening and plumping influence on boosting elasticity and refreshing your skin's appearance, which would work for those who desire to safeguard the skin from aging.

How to use:

Before use, usually wash the sponge thoroughly. We recommend plunging it in normal water and squeezing it often. If the sponge offers dry out, constantly allow it fully absorb water before putting it against your skin layer.

Carefully massage the facial skin and body inside a circular motion around, to exfoliate dead skin cells, and deep cleanse. The massaging will stimulate exhausted epidermis & encourage epidermis renewal. Soap or cleansing solution could be placed into the sponge if desired but isn't essential.

Your sponge should last almost a year, but once it begins to look tired, or begins to breakdown. Please replace it. The better treatment you require of the sponge, the a lot longer it'll last.

Konjac Face Sponge - Folks from France Pink Clay

An ideal Konjac Sponge for all those exceptional extremes from the components of air-con, excess sun exposure, and central heating. Pure French Red Clay softly purifies even the most delicate epidermis and includes a softening and plumping effect on boosting elasticity and refreshing your skin's appearance.

How to use:

Before use, perpetually wash the sponge thoroughly. We recommend plunging it in normal water and squeezing it often. If the sponge provides dry out, usually allow it fully absorb water before putting it against your skin layer.

Softly massage the facial skin and body within a circular motion around, to exfoliate dead skin cells, and deep cleanse. The massaging will stimulate exhausted epidermis & encourage epidermis renewal. Soap or cleansing solution could be placed into the sponge if desired but isn't essential.

Your sponge should last almost a year, but once it begins to look tired, or begins to breakdown. Please replace it. The better treatment you bring of the sponge, the a lot longer it'll last.

Konjac Face Sponge - Lavender

Lavender can be an all-natural relaxant and detoxifier with impressive recovery capabilities. This beautiful blossom has strong skills to relax and reduce stress and anxious tension, rendering it perfect for soothing skin treatment.

How to use:

Before use, constantly wash the sponge thoroughly. We recommend plunging it in normal water and squeezing it often. If the sponge offers dry out, perpetually allow it fully absorb water before putting it against your skin layer.

Lightly massage the facial skin and body inside a circular motion around to exfoliate dead skin cells and deep cleanse. The massaging will stimulate exhausted epidermis & encourage epidermis renewal. Soap or cleansing solution could be placed into the sponge if desired but isn't essential.

Your sponge should last almost a year, but once it begins to look tired, or begins to breakdown. Please replace it.

The better treatment you choose of the sponge, the a lot longer it'll last.

Chapter 4

Gua-Sha: The DIY Beauty Tool for An Inside-Out Glow

Self-care and skincare may actually move together; Eva Ramirez explores the historic ritual of Gua-sha and just how it could promote medical health insurance and radiance from within.

Gua-sha (pronounced gwa-sha) is definitely an old self-care practice within traditional Chinese medicine whenever a tool, usually produced from jade, bone or horn, is scraped over the skin to redirect energy stream. Using this method, stagnant energy is divided, reducing irritation, increasing blood flow, and stimulating the lymphatic system to advertise healing in the body. It's an easy but demanding technique that's used for a long time and years to take care of problems such as for example fever, muscle pain, and pressure, swelling, chronic coughs, sinusitis, and migraines.

Self-care is a center point of Chinese medication, where

it really is named Yang Sheng (healthy life), and traditionally, Gua-sha was practiced in the home. As is merely how numerous historical wellness customs, it has become a lot more popular under western culture. Much like cupping or acupressure, many acupuncturists and professionals offer Gua-sha massage therapy as a remedy in their centers. Like an athletics therapeutic massage, but having a prop, it really is carried out with medium to extreme pressure around a person's neck, legs, and arms, honing in on whichever areas specifically is in need of attention. The friction from your repeated strokes leads to scary-looking bruising and inflammation that may last for times after treatment.

Why Should We Make Dry Body Cleaning a normal Habit

Just what does this want to do with beauty and skincare? Well, a gentler version from the Gua-sha technique works just like a miracle when applied on the facial skin. There's no need to go to a therapist because everything, in regards to your skin, continues to be looked after through your regular everyday skincare.

Can A Reiki Face Heal YOUR SKIN Layer?

All you have to get is a Gua-sha tool, and in regards to a minute every day to see instant results and long-term benefits. Studies also show that day-by-day ritual enhances microcirculation by up to 400%, reduces wrinkles, rejuvenates, tones and smoothens skin, boosts collagen, combats pigmentation, dark circles, and puffy eyes, defines jawlines as well as decongests the sinuses. It's literally like rubbing your path to healthier, glower skin. Because it primarily works through the within out, you'll also notice a release of tension and relaxing of facial muscles, in the event that you clench your jaw at night time it's a sensible way to ease any soreness every day. In the event that you often get eye twitches from insomnia or stress, holding the Gua-sha over your eyes with gentle pressure may also support relieve and relax the muscles.

To be certain you're using the proper tools for the task, it's easier to get yourself a Gua-sha made of jade. Aside from looking beautiful on your own dresser, this green rock is revered due to its air-con properties; steering clear of anything produced from bone and horn for apparent factors; it's also sensible to avoid cheaper alternatives that may be created from acrylic or additional artificial chemicals that may irritate your skin layer. Applying facial oil before massaging might help the stone to glide easier while moisturizing your skin layer too.

Katie Brindle is a Chinese medicine specialist and creator of Hayo'u, an all-natural medical health insurance and skincare brand situated in the uk. Hayo'u makes the self-treatment element of Chinese medication accessible and approachable with simple daily rituals and useful techniques. They offer the equipment, such as for example their Gua-sha, which is usually carved from traditional Xiuyan Jade and carries a velvet pouch (ideal for traveling) aswell as short easy-to-follow videos to have the ability to perfect the ritual in the home.

Weather practice may be the initial thing to do like an early morning ritual or as an evening wind-down to remove the day's stress from your face, this mindful beauty practice is usually meditative and relaxing.

Chapter 5

Beauty Restored - The Advantages of Face Gua-Sha

Transform your tone with these facial massage therapy techniques. You are able to tell a whole lot about someone by merely looking at their face, not merely the manifestation of their pulling or the immediate feel they may be actually. But health and fitness will also be written on see your face, and that's because, according to Chinese medication, your beauty is definitely an external representation of the internal health.

So our beauty routines are definite improvements to your overall health. Our creator and resident physician, Katie, has captured the substance of a lot of a long time of Chinese wisdom into some powerful one-minute rituals. Quick and straightforward to accomplish, they are able to fit neatly into our modern lives, offering a transformative approach to health and fitness, subsequently providing you a healthy, glowing, and radiant tone.

Recreate your beauty

We're likely to demonstrate three iconic Chinese approaches for improving your appearance, we've processed them, and which means they may be done in mere in regards to a minute each.

They may be Àn-fa (press-hold) Gua-Sha (press stroke) and Acupressure (press-turn).

It's been within the Chinese facial massage therapy for a lot of years and revered due to its restorative, chilling properties.

Our studies showed that 82% of women found an instantaneous, positive impact after just one single minute useful.

·   Àn-fa

In this technique, you will need to press and support the jade Beauty RestorerTM over your face; press-holding the jade may reduce swelling and increase lymphatic drainage.

You may take the sweetness RestorerTM around the eyes to ease fatigue, alleviate eyesight bags, puffy eye, or twitching eyes muscles. You can also utilize the jade tool over any region to help ease stress-related symptoms such as for example headaches, flushing, epidermis circumstances, and throbbing temples.

· Gua-Sha

Gua-Sha is an easy press and heart stroke technique along the curves of this person, as shown. This beauty treatment continues to be used across Asia for a lot of years. It's renowned due to its unique capacity to increase blood circulation under your skin layer, bringing in nourishment and improving collagen.

So, instead of applying a cream or serum to improve your skin layer from the surface, you're activating your body to nourish your skin layer in an even more profound and meaningful way. This self-massage technique has shown in studies to boost circulation by 400%. It stimulates the dermis to assist collagen creation, manipulating parts of stress to relax cosmetic muscles, exponentially raises bloodstream and lymphatic movement. All this leads to a brighter, healthier, more radiant tone.

·   Acupressure

Activating acupressure factors on your face is an excellent way to assist your organs internally. Chinese medication recognizes that cosmetic beauty is usually from your organisms, this way the health of your overall health is shown for the reason of that person.

Chapter 6

What are the Advantages of Gua-Sha?

Gua-sha may reduce swelling, so it's often used to deal with illnesses that cause chronic pain, such as for example arthritis and fibromyalgia, aswell as those that bring about muscle and joint pain.

Gua-sha may possibly also relieve symptoms of other conditions like:

1. Hepatitis B

Hepatitis B is a viral contamination that triggers liver organ inflammation, liver harm, and liver organ scarring. Research demonstrates gua-sha may reduce persistent liver inflammation.

A trusted research study followed up a man with high liver enzymes, a sign of liver irritation; he was offered gua-sha medication, and after 48 hours of treatment, he experienced a reduction in liver organ enzymes. However, some experts also believe that gua-sha can improve liver swelling, thus decreasing the likelihood of liver harm. More research is underway.

2. Migraine headaches

In case your migraines usually do not relieve you after taking "over-the-counter medications," gua-sha might help. A report from a reliable source implies that a 72-year-old female dealing with chronic headaches received gua-sha a lot more than 2 weeks, and her migraines relieved during this time period, suggesting that this ancient curing technique could be an efficient fix for problems.

3. Breast engorgement

Breast engorgement is a problem experienced by many breastfeeding women, i.e., when the chest is overfilled with dairy, this usually occurs in the first weeks of breastfeeding. The mother's breast becomes inflamed and painful, rendering it difficult for babies to latch. However, this usually is a short-term condition.

Study demonstrates women receive gua-sha from the very next day after expecting until departing a healthcare facility; a healthcare facility adopted the gua-sha medication on women in the weeks after expecting, and they found that much-experienced relief of engorgement, breasts fullness, and pain, this managed to get easier to allow them to breastfeed.

4. Neck pain

Gua-sha technique in addition has been became an effective fix for chronic throat pain. To consider the potency of therapy, 48 research participants were placed into two organizations; one group was offered gua-sha, as well as the additional used a thermal heat pad to deal with throat pain. After a week, people who received gua-sha reported less pain compared to the group that didn't receive gua-sha.

5. Tourette syndrome

Tourette symptoms involve involuntary motions such as

for example face tics, neck clearing, and vocal outbursts. Associated with a person, gua-sha in conjunction with various other therapies may possess help to reduce symptoms of Tourette in the analysis participant.

The analysis involved a 33-year-old male who had Tourette syndrome at age 9; he received acupuncture, natural herbs, gua-sha, and altered his lifestyle, his symptoms relieved by 70 percent. Despite the fact that this man got positive results, further research is essential.

6. Pre-menopausal syndrome

Pre-menopausal occurs as women near menopause. Symptoms include:

- Insomnia.

- Irregular periods.

- Anxiety.

- Fatigue.

- hot flashes

Studies, however, show that gua-sha may reduce premenopausal symptoms in a few women. The analysis examined 80 women with premenopausal symptoms. The procedure group received 15 tiny gua-sha treatments once weekly, as well as standard therapy for eight weeks. The control group only received regular therapy.

Upon completion of the analysis, the involvement group reported an increased reduction of symptoms such as for example insomnia, anxiety, exhaustion, headaches, and hot flashes compared to the control group.

Experts believe gua-sha therapy may be considered a safe, effective treatment for these symptoms.

Will Gua-Sha have UNWANTED EFFECTS?

As an all-natural healing treatment, gua-sha is safe. It's not reported to be unpleasant, however the procedure may change the looks of your skin layer since it entails massaging or scraping epidermis having a massage therapy tool, tiny arteries referred to as capillaries near to the surface of your skin layer can burst; this might lead to epidermis bruising and small loss of blood. Bruising usually disappears in a few days.

A lot of people also experience short-term indentation of their epidermis after a gua-sha treatment. Three necessary precautions will be the following:

·   If any bleeding occurs, there's also the opportunity of moving blood-borne illnesses with gua-sha therapy, so technicians must disinfect their tools after each person.

·   Avoid this technique if you've acquired any surgery in the last six weeks.

Individuals who are taking bloodstream thinners or have clotting disorders aren't suitable applicants for gua-sha.

Chapter 7

How to do Gua-Sha for Face in 11 Simple Actions

Once I first noticed it's likely you have a Gua-Sha for face and throat, I have been amazed. I've been a lover of the historical treatment but didn't recognize that there's a face version.

Great things about Face Gua-Sha

Gua-Sha, for the facial skin and neck, is known as the Eastern Botox (or Eastern Facelift). This traditional Chinese medication treatment, when placed on the facial skin, gets the next results:

·   Support your sagging facial muscles.

·   Smoothens your skin layer and reduces the looks of lines and wrinkles on see your face.

·   Improves dark circles and handbags beneath the eye (the sort you obtain from advancing generation).

·	Lightens age and additional epidermis discolorations.

·	Your tone gets rosier and more radiant.

·	Helps remove acne, rosacea, and other epidermis diseases oyour face

I have a first-hand reference to everything around the list apart from the last, and although we are used to expecting great results because of my positive encounters with body Gua-Sha, I have been nonetheless amazed to start out to see the improvements on my face.

I'd halted taking Glutathione and Grape Seed, but after a week or two of face Gua-Sha, my face includes a clearness and radiance that I'd just generally possess while on those supplements.

How it operates

As discussed above, Gua-Sha is identified to end up being the age-old practice which involves the scraping movements all over the surface of ones body having a smooth-edged tool: it really is hard enough to boost petechial, reddish marks that typically transmit a Gua-Sha therapy program.

Gua-Sha scraping

Face Gua-Sha will be a lot much milder but has got the same scraping action along your skin layer; as your skin layer is usually scraped, the layers of your skin layer are activated, and stagnant lymph that creates puffiness is usually relocated and cleared from the machine; poisons will also be released, creating a brighter appearance and finally, the massaging action relaxes anxious muscles that wrinkles provide.

Eastern Botox in 11 Steps

Many reminders for beginners:

·   Don't utilize the same heavy pressure that you have when scraping the body. As a result of this to work, you should employ only light-weight. The facial skin is more delicate than the areas of the body.

· We are moving stagnant lymph from our face. We will drain this out via the proper and remaining lymphatic ducts. They will be the areas among your collarbones.

· All our (light) scraping movements will be upwards. Remember; we are countering sagging, so we can not ever make any downward actions. The only exclusion may be the finished part if we do the dumping in the lymphatic ducts highlighted above.

Cosmetic Gua-sha

Now here would be the general actions you are able to do like a newbie:

· Third Vision: Heart stroke from the guts of the eyebrows or even more to your hairline. This region activates curing.

· Lower forehead: Sweep from your guts from the forehead above your eyebrows venturing out to your temples.

· Under eyebrow: Make use of the curved part of

your gua-sha tool to scrape the spot underneath your eyebrow and above your eye. Adhere to the bone from the brow.

·   Under the attention: Slowly and lightly stroke the spot where your vision bags typically show; start through the medial side of the nasal and rise to your temple. Imagine moving the stagnant lymph from the guts of this person up to the temple and entirely towards the hairline.

·   Cheek: Do the same sweeping movement for the cheek area. Proceed in the medial side of the nasal, across your cheek, or even more again to the guts of the ear.

·   Jaws: Do the same for the jaws again, sweeping the lymph upwards to your ear.

·   Chin: Sweep from the guts of this person, under your lower lip, and to the earlobe.

·   Under chin: Scrape from your soft field under your chin to underneath of the hearing.

·   Throat: Finally, it's time and energy to scrape from

your own jaw and earlobe because of the center of the collarbone.

The very best sweep: Collect all of the lymph you've moved aside from the facial skin and dumped it to your lymphatic drainage, sweep through the guts of the forehead right under your hairline, because of your temple, because of your hearing until you reach your throat and terminus area. Do often for any clean sweep.

Chapter 8

How to Give Yourself the Best Gua-Sha Face at Home

What exactly does gua-sha do?

Gua-sha pre-dates acupuncture; the heart stroke design used, awakens the meridian lines (life force route) to activate the body's natural curing abilities. For your skin layer, gua-sha stimulates collagen creation (power in cells); it sculpts and shades the facial skin kind, allowing irritation to drain and muscles to become free from pressure - permitting them to create their supportive careers properly. Also, it can help your skin get back to its most radiant condition as blood flow is usually increased, sending nutrition to areas that may have already been starved due to blockage.

Gua-Sha's impact is a lot more than epidermis deep; as the meridian lines are enlivened, organs just like the belly, liver, spleen, center, and kidneys also get a great advantage. Coping with gua-sha tools over the spot from the facial skin from the kidneys allows them to use at ideal capacity.

What exactly are the huge benefits?

·   Bears nutrient-rich and oxygenated bloodstream (food for the cells) to your skin layer and tissues

·   Drains lymph liquid (which is often loaded with poisons and spend) from your cells to become cleansed

·   Eliminates or considerably reduces wrinkles

·   Treats and aids in preventing sagging epidermis (elevates and tightens your skin layer)

·   Aids in removing dark circles round the eyes

·   Aids in divorce and liberating your skin layer from shaded areas and hyper-pigmentation

- Brightens the complexion

- Exceedingly rates the curing period of breakouts and acne, helping these epidermis issues overall

- Has the capability to heal and relieve rosacea

- Supports product penetration

- Goodies TMJ disorder and migraines

- Is an alternative solution to shots and face-lift surgery (when used frequently in the home or when obtaining treatments from a qualified practitioner)

How will you select a Gua-sha Tool?

Gua-sha tools can be found in a range of different designs, sizes, and forms; some devices are created from pet bone and horn, some from gemstones (like jade or increased quartz), and several professionals utilize the Chinese soup spoons. I've even seen the cover of the cup jar (one with curved and soft sides) within a pinch.

Trending at this time is usually increased quartz and jade; jade established fact for inviting serenity and purity, aswell as promoting fertility, balance, and deep recovery. Rose quartz established fact for restoring tranquillity deep in to the heart. It is the stone of universal love and promotes unconditional caring and compassion.

Choosing your gua-sha rock is related to choosing a crystal or gemstone. When you can select it out personally, please do that. Choose it up, experience it, observe its feels in the hands. See which catches your attention - if the foremost is sparkling a little more for you personally than others, prefer it!

What's the main element to a rewarding practice?

Regularity may be the key; to maintain a flourishing and keep maintaining a sound body, we regularly nourish ourselves with normal water, rest, clean eating, and motion. Likewise, training gua-sha frequently will prove best suited. The body doesn't thrive if we are oscillating to either extreme - the guts is always best suited.

Since you will find 20 liters of liquid that circulate through the body each day (and around three liters from the fluid becomes lymph liquid), it is rather supportive to the body to produce this practice in to the daily routine. However, getting gua-sha into the daily life every day could be challenging, but carving out a fantastic short amount of time a few days weekly is active (even if it's only two minutes). You might spot the body starting to crave these occasions of self-care.

Pressure and purpose will also be essential to your practice; the touch ought to be very soft, and you'll test out different degrees of pressure. But always sweep the gua-sha rock across your face in specific movements. The lighter the touches, the bigger you are assisting the lymph liquid, and with a rise of pressure, know you're engaging in muscle. Please be cautious that you should not bruise or cause distress.

How will you prep your skin layer?

Using a clean face and clean hands, mist generously

having a hydrosol (I love True Botanicals Renew Nutrient Mist, OSEA's Sea Vitamin Boost or Heritage Store's Rose Water), then apply facial oil (I love True Botanicals Renew Radiance Oil, OSEA's Undaria Argan Oil or Shiva Rose face oil) around see your face and neck; using the fundamental oil left around the hands, grease up your gua-sha tool. Then, start - all while taking deep, cleansing breaths.

How will you perform Gua-sha?

Cleanse Face and Hands - After blow drying the facial skin using a clean washcloth, generously mist see your face. The hydrosol is a superb vehicle to use the fundamental oil - which you'll apply next - deep in to the epidermis, especially towards the layers that want nourishment and hydration. (Suggestion: I only use my washcloth once, and it switches into the hamper. When you have issues with breakouts, it's best never to reuse cosmetic towels before cleaning. Bacteria can transfer again on your skin.)

Apply Facial - Gas (from 4-10 drops), within the facial

skin and throat; apply gas starting within the forehead and moving down in direction of draining lymph liquid. This activates motion in epidermis and cells, and it's an excellent prep prior to the gua-sha.

Warm Gua-Sha Tool - slightly by rubbing it between your hands. This also greases the tool up just a little such that it doesn't draw on your own skin layer in the areas that didn't receive as much gas.

Sweep Up Your GUITAR NECK On Both Edges - Sweep very softly over your Adam's apple; that is even more of an instant sweep to activate your REN collection. (The REN route in Chinese medication collects the body's yin energy, goodies and the problems from the stomach, chest, neck, mind, and face.)

Sweep Under Your Chin - from the guts of that person away to your earlobe, keeping your tool smooth. If you'd like, support the epidermis under your chin together with your additional thumb as you glide these devices back to your earlobe in the contrary direction.

Sweep FROM YOUR Centre OF THE Chin Over Your Jawline - again toward your earlobe, you are able to gently jiggle in the hearing to encourage the liquid to drain down the throat towards the lymph nodes in the bottom, just above your collarbone.

Sweep Underneath Your Cheekbone - really picking up significant amounts of liquid that's commonly stored here, and direct it toward your hairline. You are able to lightly jiggle your tool on the hairline.

Sweep over Your Cheekbones - finishing in the hairline.

Very Gently Sweep Under Your Eye - I love sweeping through the area of the attention relocating toward the midline; the muscle agreements with this path as well as the lymph offers little streams moving down from the attention entirely from the inner corner from the focus on the outer part. But if it appears better to sweep from the inside edge from the care towards the hairline, do that - that is an even more traditional path for gua-sha.

Sweep AROUND THE Eyebrow Out Toward The Hairline OR EVEN MORE FROM YOUR OWN Brow Bone - (in the forehead) finishing on the hairline; when you sweep up, take action in tiny areas, moving along the eyebrow in three to five sections.

Sweep from the middle of your Eyebrows over another Eye or even more towards the Hairline - Detect in case your clairvoyance seems more activated on third stroke

Sweep THROUGH THE Centre FROM THE Forehead Out To The Hairline - Among the best techniques hails from Britta Plug of Britta Beauty in NYC. She sweeps from the guts from the forehead and doesn't touch the hairline and proceeds in to the locks, behind the hearing and down the throat. It feels divine.)

Now Caress the Other Part of this Person - starting again together with your neck and working through the steps.

Glide Down The Medial Side - When you've completed the other facet of see your face, finish the task by sweeping down the throat to assist with enduring drainage. Keep carefully the tool very toned and hug underneath your jawbone, gently sweep down the throat towards the collarbone.

Essential ideas to help make nearly all your practice:

·   I would recommend sweeping each area at minimal 3x; for extended practice, sweep up to 10 times.

·   Maintain your tool level to your skin layer (about 15 degrees) instead of getting the benefit of the tool at 90 degrees to your skin layer.

·   Whenever your tool begins to pull or draw on your own skin layer, devote a bit more gas for an improved slide.

·   Have fun trying out which aspect and type of the tool best suit your face. Remember, what feels correct for you personally, may appear unique of how it seems in videos.

How often should i practice Gua-sha?

I would suggest incorporating gua-sha in to the self-care program daily, however when it begins to feel like an activity, have a rest.

Precisely what does it feel like?

Gua-sha is also known as very relaxing, mainly when the

pressure is only right, usage adoring, and mild strokes; be intentional within your touch. It'll feel just like you are sweeping the gua-sha on the stunning, soft skin of the infant.

You may feel the fluids moving, which is fantastic! You may feel your skin layer becoming alive or as if it's returning and waking up. I often time start the medication in the still left, since it is reported to be the medial side from the feminine energy, which is more utilized at receiving. I've remarked that when the rest of the team of this person gets, it primes the proper part to be more responsive.

Just how much gua-sha is an excessive amount of?

Avoid gua-sha in the event that you merely received injections. Botox requires at least a fortnight staying.

Avoid gua-sha over cystic acne, pimples, and start lesions, since it is only going to irritate contaminated areas, but gua-sha is quite beneficial inside the breakout. Draining below the breakout allows the lymph to move poisons towards the lymph nodes. That is where spend will exist cleansed prior to the period for the circulatory system to nourish the body.

Repeat each heart stroke inside the same region, only ten occasions. If you're repeating the sweeping way too many instances, you might cause an excessive amount of activation. Liquids are potent; you could finish off moving an excessive amount of spend at onetime, causing detoxification symptoms (such as for example dizziness or emotions of decreasing using the flu).

Chapter 9

CELLULITE

Cellulite usually starts round the hips and thighs and mostly along the yang meridians; the place to start is usually the Gall Bladder, small yang meridian, perhaps as the Qi in the Gall Bladder is usually less than in the other yang meridians. Cellulite explains the dimpling of your skin layer, triggered from the protrusion of subcutaneous extra fat in to the dermis, creating an undulating junction in the middle of your epidermis and subcutaneous adipose cells.

The Spleen nourishes muscle and fat, as well as the function from the Spleen is to distribute fat evenly through the body, especially in the periphery. Regarding cellulite, the excess fat distribution is affected, and fat seems to stagnate without circulation in a few regions of your body. So, on normally the one hand, there is without a doubt excess fat, and on the additional, there is without a doubt poor circulation from it. This creates the picture of imbalance explained above.

However, we likewise have the problem in the meridian along which this problem occurs - that may be Gall Bladder but may also be Urinary Bladder and even Stomach, regarding the patient. So both Spleen as well as the affected meridians need to be good balanced.

Body Acupuncture Treatment

Example - cellulite around the lateral part of thighs

· Gall Bladder - UB 19 (Back-Shu stage), GB 37 (Luo level).

· Spleen - UB 20 (Back-Shu period), St 40 (Luo place).

· Local needles and moving cup massage.

· Two sessions weekly, 8-10 sessions altogether.

This treatment principle can be employed on affected meridian. For example, for the Bladder meridian - you should use UB 28 (the Back-Shu position, to improve the function) and UB 58 (the Luo-connecting point of yang meridian, to tonify the yang and reduce the yin aspect).

Local treatment is fairly useful if performed good. Patients sometimes want to hurry through the neighborhood process because cupping massage therapy isn't so pleasant - it's necessary to show patience while taking this treatment.

Special local therapy

If the affected area is privately along the Gall Bladder meridian, this treatment ought to be achieved in two halves, with the average person lying using one side 1st and having all of the tiny needles and cupping; then thrilled the various other aspect and obtaining the same treatment.

·   Lying privately, factors on your own body - UB 18, UB 20, St 40, GB 37.

·   At exactly the same time, about 10 to 15 local tiny needles around the cellulite (15-20 cm tiny needles of 0.20 mm gauge) are inserted wholly and perpendicularly, at about 3 cm distance in one another.

· Both body needles and local needles are remaining in situ for 20 minutes.

· After all the needles are removed, apply St John's wort oil sparingly on the spot of cellulite. Usually, do not overdo this, as it'll reduce friction for the massage therapy.

· Place a large cup (for a specific cellulite glass) at the reduced end from the thigh using an open fire for creating vacuum pressure, and slip the container along the spot before epidermis becomes quite red. This technique is fairly unpleasant for the average person, and if very sore, in that case your vacuum could possibly be reduced. The massage therapy takes in regards to a minute.

· The specific may remark that this legs feel very light following a treatment.

· Treatment is administered twice regularly, for 8-10 times like a course.

What can the average person do in the home?

As cellulite is stagnation of fat, the average person can execute a large amount of things in the home in order to avoid its formation and to improve circulation.

·   Foods that creates fat tissue in the body are; fatty foods, fatty dairy food (low-fat dairy food could be consumed in smaller amounts), processed sugars, and sugar (though wholemeal, fruits, sugars, and honey are fine). These food types ought to be prevented.

·   When fat tissue becomes too thicker, the blood flow is affected. It really is, therefore, crucial that the average person drinks normal water regularly and throughout the day - the regularity is more important compared to the number consumed. Hot water surpasses cool, which is impressive how quickly patients come to enjoying hot water.

·   Finally, they need to work daily around the cellulite, massaging it with very soft spiky toners and pummelling these areas to break the stagnation. Seated cross-legged to the floor and moving sideways and ahead and back this position, resulting in friction on parts of cellulite ('bum walking'), for quarter-hour every day in the comfort of their residence is definitely an additional solution to greatly help improve blood flow.

Gua-Sha MASSAGE THERAPY Cellulite Singapore

Looking for cure for the unequal, lumpy epidermis on your own hips, thighs, or buttocks? The Gua-Sha Massage therapy Cellulite brings everything towards the desk; you don't need to exist ashamed of the body appearance any more.

·   Meet Gua-Sha: The Cellulite Remover

Gua-Sha massage therapy is a therapy technique used to deal with several ailments; these include pains and aches, strains, lumbar stress, arthritis rheumatoid, and heart stroke.   The activation of blood flow triggers its therapeutic impact; this relieves bloodstream stagnation.

Moreover, the Gua-Sha Massage Cellulite eliminates or reduces the introduction of cellulite in the body.

Advantages of Gua-Sha:

·   Improves hydration levels.

·   Relieves stress.

·   Gets gone or reduces Cellulite.

·   Relaxes face muscles.

·   Improves blood flow etc.

Gua-Sha MASSAGE THERAPY Treatment:

Your skin layer is oily, and a Gua-Sha device is gently utilized to scrape over the top of affected area; this promotes breakage of surface adhesion, increases circulation, and enhances lymph drainage and firmness; in addition, it solves the issues of fats cells and encourages a smoother appearance.

Gua-Sha can be executed on any section of the body. Maybe it's performed on section of the body, even within the facial skin. It can benefit to relax your skin layer and improve the blood flow in the facial skin and improve collagen creation; it gets your skin layer look more radiant and reduces lines and wrinkles.

Also, people utilize massage techniques or dry brushing to remove cellulite. The triggering of cells manually really helps to improve blood flow and in addition reduces adipose tissue, specifically in keeping energies like unwanted weight. Thus, it boosts skin radiance.

Acknowledgements

The Glory of this book success goes to God Almighty and my beautiful Family, Fans, Readers & well-wishers, Customers, and Friends for their endless support and encouragement.